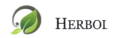 

Homemade Health

Anke Bialas

Homemade Health

HOME REMEDIES YOUR GRANDMOTHER KNEW
SIMPLE & EFFECTIVE TREATMENTS FROM THE PANTRY

Anke Bialas

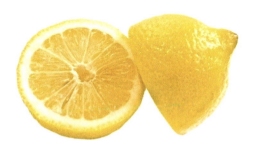

Natator

Publishing

ISBN 9780980766851

First published in Australia, 2012 by Natator Publishing
Images under license by Depositphotos

National Library of Australia Cataloguing-in-Publication entry

Bialas, Anke, 1968-
Homemade health: home remedies your
grandmother knew - simple & effective treatments from the pantry /
Anke Bialas.
ISBN: 9780980766851 (pbk.)
Bialas, Anke, 1968- Herbology at home.
Herbs--Therapeutic use.
Traditional medicine.
Self-care, Health.
Dewey Number: 610

This book is intended as an educational reference guide only, not a medical manual. The information given here is designed to help make informed decisions about your health. It is not intended as a substitute for any treatment that may have been prescribed by your medical professional. If you suspect you have a medical problem, we urge you to seek professional help. The author takes no responsibility for the misinterpretation and deliberate or accidental misuse of the information presented in this book, on the website and on any published Herbology material.

Let food be thy medicine and medicine be thy food.

Hippocrates 460-377BC

Thank You ....

....to my wonderful husband, without whom the Herbology seed would never have been sown.

....to contributors from far and wide.

There have been many helpful suggestions by the online community that follows *Herbology At Home* but there are a few people I'd like to single out for their continued support and contributions.

Leslie Postin
Renée Hotschilt
Sonya Lowe
Julie Collier
Amanda McCamley
Betheny
Paul Watson
Debs Cook
Suzie Eisfelder

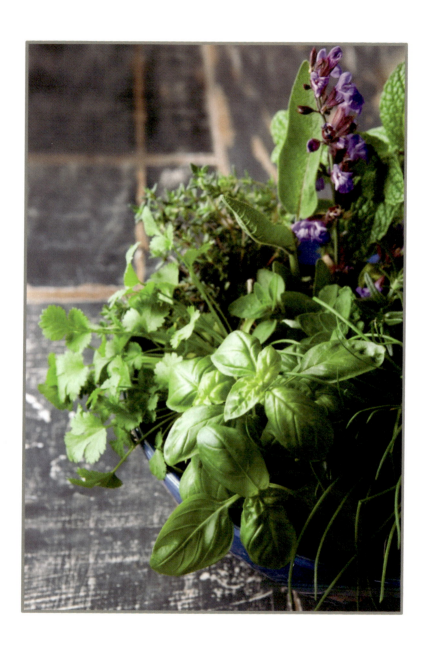

Contents

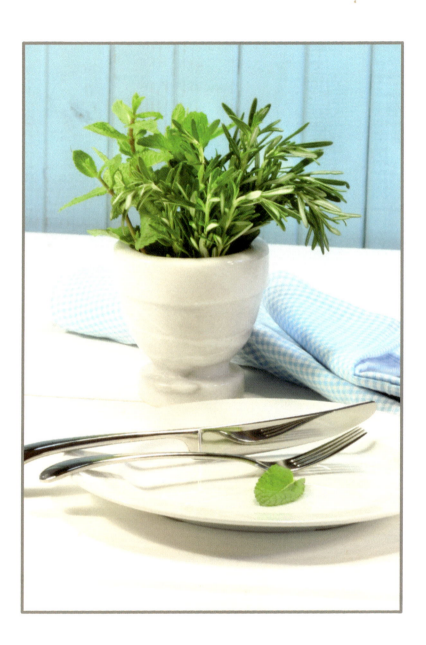

Introduction

Who doesn't have at least one childhood memory of Mum or Grandma taking something from the pantry to ease discomfort caused by an everyday mishap? Milk, butter, water, and aloe vera were common treatments for burns. Onions and garlic emerged for all manner of emergencies from toothaches to insect bites. Chamomile tea eased the tummy and helped a teething infant sleep. We trusted them completely and did not question their cures.

Old world remedies are back in favour. After a long time of relying on products from the drugstore people now prefer to go back to natural, time honoured treatments for minor ailments and injuries.

In *Homemade Health* I have translated many old German remedies I grew up with. There have also been a number of contributions from loyal Herbology readers who came forward when I put out the word about this project.

Some of the remedies you will find to be more amusing than practical, although they may well work. I have not included any of the more questionable or downright dangerous practices that were popular a few hundred years ago, regardless of whether they work or not. Having said that, I still need to make the necessary disclaimer that the information given here is designed to help make informed decisions about your health. It is not intended as a substitute for any treatment that may have been prescribed by your medical professional.

That out of the way, please enjoy *Homemade Health* as it is intended, from acne to warts – natural, old world remedies from the pantry. Treat your family's minor ailments with traditional folk remedies your grandmother knew and used.

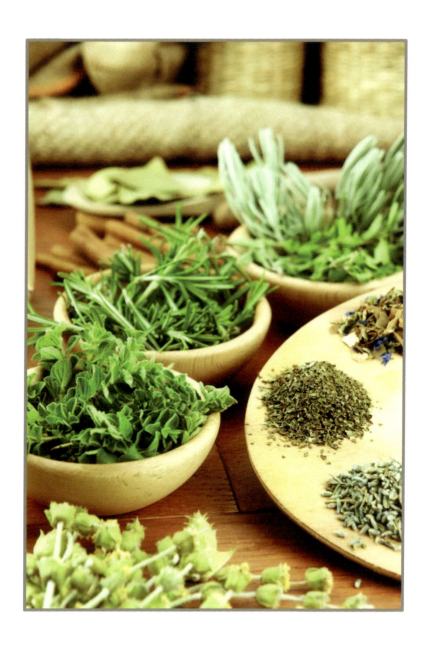

Kitchen Herbs Are Medicine Too

DO YOU HAVE THESE IN YOUR KITCHEN?

- **Basil** (*Ocimum basilicum*)
- **Cloves** (*Syzygium aromaticum*)
- **Garlic** (*Allium sativum*)
- **Nutmeg** (*Myristica frayrans*)
- **Oats** (*Avena sativa*)
- **Rosemary** (*Rosmarinus officinalis*)
- **Sage** (*Salvia officinalis*)
- **Thyme** (*Thymus vulgaris*)

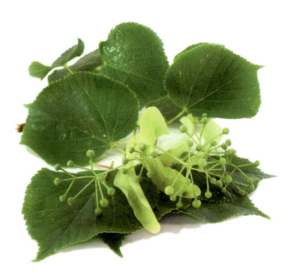

LINDEN
Tilia cordata

Have you ever wondered what came first – a combination of food with herb because of complementing flavours, or a combination of food with herb for health benefits?

I have been thinking about this one a bit recently. We associate a rich pork roast with sage, Eastern Europeans wouldn't dream of eating their cabbage without caraway, winter savoury is linked to beans and if you are a fan of goose then adding mugwort is a must. We associate those flavours but the herbs in question each help with the digestion of the foods involved. Sage and mugwort cut through the fattiness and richness, caraway and winter savoury combat the "windy" consequences of eating cabbage and beans. So which came first?

Did our ancestors somewhere down the track realise that sage made them feel better after eating rich, fatty meat dishes? Or was that a side effect of pairing the foods purely based on taste? Oh, and wasn't Mother Nature wonderful for designing it this way?

At a time when there were no health food stores and online herb suppliers not everyone had access to medicinal herbs. Or did they? People distinguish between medicinal and culinary herbs but really, culinary herbs *ARE* medicinal as well. So what do you do when you can't get what you want? You make do with what you do have.

Shops and markets are full of herbs meant for the kitchen and these herbs can be used to stock your home pharmacy. I won't go through all the commonly used culinary herbs, their uses and healing properties, but here are a few to spark your interest.

BASIL (ocimum basilicum)

Favoured by the Italians, basil quickly loses it volatile oils and flavour so it is best added at the end of the cooking process. There are so many culinary uses for Basil and it is great combined with tomato. Medicinally, basil is used to combat stress, tension and nervous indigestion. It is cooling to the body and a natural mood enhancer.

CLOVES (Syzygium aromaticum)

Cloves are often associated with Mexican and Indian cuisine and old recipes that grandma used to make. Medicinally, clove oil is a well known (if pungent) remedy for toothache. It is an analgesic with powerful germicidal properties. Cloves have been known to reduce fever. Often prepared as a decoction or infusion it can be made more palatable by adding cinnamon and apple peel.

GARLIC (Allium sativum)

Garlic has been helping people for centuries. A veritable powerhouse of active ingredients which are reported to ease an A-Z of ailments and treating high blood pressure is one of the health issues on this list. It has long been said that if fresh garlic is regularly included in ones daily diet, it would ease hypertension. What does that mean in practical terms? Well, I interpret it to mean that garlic is great for you anyway for many reasons including regulating your blood pressure. But if you have a problem with high blood pressure you may now have a natural way of reducing your reliance on blood pressure medication as well. Of course, do not stop taking prescribed medication without first consulting your doctor.

NUTMEG (Myristica fragrans)

Very little nutmeg is needed to lend its slightly sweet, spicy flavour to milk based sauces, or in brewed drinks like eggnog, mulled wine, and mulled cider. Medicinally, it is used to treat nausea, vomiting, and indigestion. Large doses of nutmeg can be toxic.

OATS (Avena sativa)

Oats are a well known staple on the breakfast table. Whether it is oatmeal which is popular in the US or porridge in the UK, oats and oat products are well known and well loved all over the world. Particularly in cold weather, oats are often eaten to generate inner warmth and slow-release energy which helps in the treatment of colds and chills.

The whole plant is utilised in herbal medicine. Also known as oatstraw, it is an excellent tonic for the nervous system. Used for both physical and nervous fatigue oats are also used for general debility. Rich in minerals, vitamins, flavonoids and more it has many healing properties. Oatstraw has antidepressant and restorative properties which make a great nerve tonic and it promotes sweating. Rich in calcium, oatstraw is used to prevent or treat osteoporosis. The grains make a nutritive and antidepressant nerve tonic while oat bran reduces cholesterol levels and has antithrombotic properties. You can also find a Wild Oats remedy amongst the Bach Flower Remedies which is recommended for times of uncertainty and dissatisfaction.

Oatstraw tincture and decoctions can be used for insomnia, anxiety and depression. The decoction also makes an effective skin wash to heal skin conditions. A poultice made from the grain has long been used to treat eczema, and other skin problems.

ROSEMARY (Rosmarinus officinalis)

Rosemary is a woody, evergreen with a wonderful smell. Its flavour is often associated with many dishes from the Mediterranean. It enhances the flavours of meats, gravies, risotto dishes, and stocks beautifully. Medicinally, Rosemary is a great herb for the mind. Rosemary has been used to improve mental faculties for many hundreds of years. It contains a compound (carnosic acid) which may be of use in the treatment of neuro-degenerative diseases. Rosemary in food and as an essential oil can be used to ease headaches and it is often used to combat depression.

 ## SAGE (Salvia officinalis)

Sage is a staple in many European kitchens. Its flavour makes it a perfect pairing with meats and cheese. Of course, what could be better that a sageflavoured stuffing for your chicken roast? Medicinally, it is a virtual cure all. Sage can be used as an astringent and has antibiotic properties. It improves sluggish digestion and sage tea is excellent for a chronic cough. For centuries sage has been used by lactating mothers to dry up the milk supply when weaning a baby. The smoke from burning sage is used to cleanse and purify spaces.

 ## THYME (Thymus vulgaris)

Thymeis found widely in culinary dishes all over the world, found in many meat, tomato, and egg dishes. It is a natural expectorant which makes it an excellent remedy for throat or bronchial problems. Being a natural antiseptic, you can use the infusion to make a gargle which reduces the inflammation associated with a sore throat.

The medicinal uses of kitchen herbs seem to have been largely forgotten. Have a look around your kitchen and see what herbs and spices you use. Why not research their healing properties and find out what else you could be using them for?

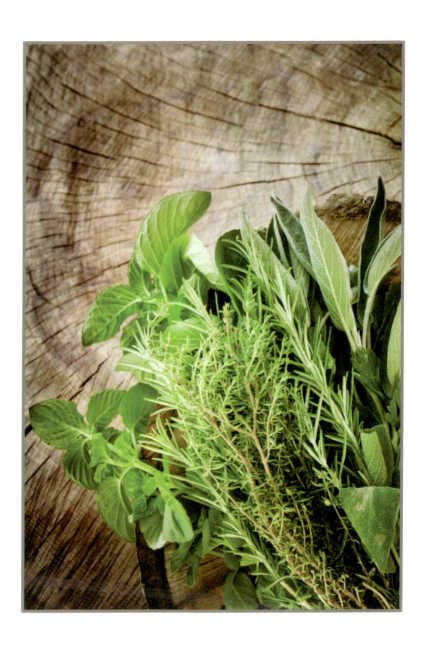

From Acne to Warts

OVER 160 HOME REMEDIES

Not so long ago, home remedies were a part of everyday life, usually the first port of call when someone felt ill. People went to their garden or kitchen pantry before going to a doctor.

Many of these simple and natural remedies are just as effective as treatments bought at the drugstore.

Try these quick and natural treatments for many common ailments.

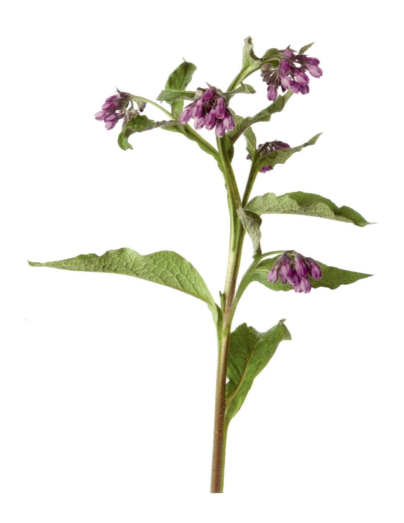

COMFREY
Symphytum officinale

ACNE

Dab fresh lemon juice on the affected area several times a day. Leave for 5 minutes then rinse with tepid water. The acid will remove excess build up or oils and clean the pores.

An infected pimple will heal much faster if you regularly dab it with arnica tincture. Never pierce an infected pimple, not even with a sterilised implement.

Plantain is an ancient herb used for health and beauty. Use plantain juice to treat problem skin and acne, topically and internally. Freshly squeezed juice can be taken 3 times daily at a dose of 1 to 2 tablespoons.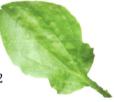

Horsetail contains astringent properties which clean and tighten pores. Make a skin wash by adding 1 handful of dried horsetail to 1 litre of boiling water, cover and steep for 15 minutes. Once cooled, use unstrained once a week.

APPETITE, LOSS OF

To stimulate the appetite drink a tea made from caraway and yarrow. Add ½ teaspoon of dried caraway and ½ teaspoon of dried yarrow to 1 cup of almost boiling water. Cover and leave for 5 minutes. Drink a cupful 30 minutes before mealtimes.

Dandelion is well known as a diuretic which aids in detoxifying the body but it also stimulates the appetite. Make a tea from 2 teaspoons of dried dandelion and 1 cup of almost boiling water, cover and leave for 15 minutes. Drink a cup in the morning and the evening.

BACK ACHE

Wash the affected area with sage tea, as hot as you can handle. One teaspoon dried sage per cup of boiling water. Cover and leave for 10 minutes. Strain before use.

A mustard plaster eases a number of back issues such as sciatica, neuralgia, joint inflammation and rheumatic pain. Quantities for the mustard paste will depend on the size of plaster required. Use a piece of cotton or linen cloth at least twice the size required. Grind mustard seeds (be aware that black are the hottest), then add 4 times as much all purpose flour and enough cool water to make a paste. Spread paste onto half the fabric, fold over, if too wet add another layer of cloth, once placed on the affected area this will increase blood circulation, perspiration and heat. Do not let the paste touch bare skin, and do not use for longer than 30 minutes. Remove and wash well with warm water.

BAD BREATH

A secret tip to treat bad breath is to chew a coffee bean. This will refresh breath very quickly.

Basil is great in treating halitosis/bad breath. Make a mouthwash by covering 1 handful of dried basil leaves with 1 cup of boiling water, cover and leave for 15 minutes. Cool, and then rinse mouth well.

Parsley chases away garlic breath when chewed fresh. A small piece of chocolate is said to have the same effect.

BEE STING

Firstly, remove the sting gently. Reduce swelling with ice or cold water. For excessive swelling see your doctor.

Moisten a cube of sugar, apply to the sting. Sugar sucks up moisture and will therefore absorb the venom; this will also reduce the itching.

Cover sting with slices of fresh onion, lemon or horseradish. If fresh garlic or onion is used to treat the sting, the pain and the swelling will lessen.

BLOOD PRESSURE

Low blood pressure can be helped by eating lots of hazelnuts and garlic.

Rosemary stimulates circulation and as such is an aide to raise blood pressure. If you suffer from low blood pressure try a herbal bath made with 100g/3 ½ oz dried rosemary infused in 3 litres/6 pints of almost boiling water, for 30 minutes. Add this infusion to your bath water.

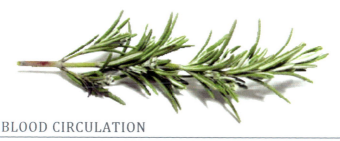

BLOOD CIRCULATION

Horse chestnuts are a well known treatment for circulation problems. A decoction of the spiky husk as well as the nuts can be added to a foot bath or full bath increases blood circulation to the area immersed and also helps with frostbite and haemorrhoids. Cover 1 kilo of chopped husks and nuts with water and bring briefly to the boil, cover and turn off heat. Leave for 30 minutes then add strained liquid to bath water.

BODY ODOUR

If body odour is a problem for you try this old remedy of taking a bath in tomato juice twice a week. For a full bath, add 500ml/1 pint of tomato juice to the water. Regular baths will banish even the strongest body odour.

COLDS

If your cold is accompanied by fevers, string cloves of garlic or small onions together and wear around your neck at bedtime. (This one may have to be tried by those of my readers who are single or whose partner loves the smell of garlic).

A decoction of ginger root eases cold & flu. Add fresh ginger root to cold water, bring to a boil then reduce to a gentle simmer for 10 minutes. Drink as hot as possible (add honey if you like) to induce sweating.

Lemon balm is also used for colds and particularly head colds. Add 1 teaspoon dried lemon balm to 1 cup of almost boiling water, cover and leave for 10 minutes to infuse. Drink twice daily.

Plantain eases coughs and acts as an expectorant. Mild but effective enough to be great for children in the form of a syrup. Plantain tea is made by adding 1 teaspoon of dried plantain to 1 cup of almost boiling water, covering and leaving for 10 minutes to infuse. Three cups of the sweetened tea should be sipped throughout the day.

Linden flowers are well known to induce perspiration and ease muscle aches. Linden flower tea has long been used in the treatment of cold and flu; it also helps ease a sore throat and coughs. Apart from that it is often drunk because it tastes great. Add 1 teaspoon dried linden flowers to 1 cup of almost boiling water, cover and leave for 10 minutes to infuse. Drink twice daily

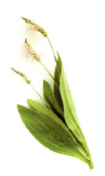

Once upon a time thyme was the herb used to treat most ailments but particularly anything related to colds and flu. Coughs were treated with steam inhalations and rubbing hot infusions directly onto the chest. Sore throats demanded the gargling of thyme tea and as an early form of aromatherapy thyme was simmered in a pot on the stove during flu season as a preventative measure, adding the many healing properties of this herb to the air. Add 1-2 teaspoons of thyme to 1 cup of almost boiling water, cover and leave to infuse for 10 minutes. Strain and drink 3 – 4 cups a day.

Fennel is great for kids. It loosens phlegm and eases cramping. A tea made from fennel seeds is a traditional remedy to ease chesty colds, coughs and tummy troubles in children. Make the tea with 1 teaspoon of freshly crushed fennel seeds and 1 cup of almost boiling water, cover and leave to steep for 5 minutes. Sip tea throughout the day. It's also popular with children to warm the seeds in milk instead of water.

COLD SORES/HERPES

The incessant itch can be eased by applying lemon balm essential oil to lip or skin.

COUGH

An old treatment for a dry cough is to use warm, unsalted potato water (water in which potatoes have been boiled), sweetened with honey as a kind of cough syrup. It does not taste very nice but is said to be very effective.

Thyme is a great foundation herb for cough treatments. Make a tea from 1 teaspoon of dried thyme, infuse for 10 minutes then strain and sweeten with honey. Coughs can also be treated by inhaling the steam from the infusion or soaking a cloth in the hot infusion and applying it directly onto the chest (not so hot as to burn yourself).

For a tickle cough try equal parts of honey and apple cider vinegar. When it strikes, let a small amount sit and slowly melt in your mouth.

Fennel loosens phlegm and eases cramping. A tea made from fennel seeds is a traditional remedy to ease chesty colds, coughs and tummy troubles in children. Make the tea with a teaspoon of freshly crushed fennel seeds and a cup of almost boiling water, cover and leave to steep for 5 minutes. Sip tea throughout the day. It's also popular with children to warm the seeds in milk instead of water.

The needles of the spruce make a good expectorant cough treatment. To make a cough syrup alternate layers of young shoots with layers of sugar. Fill a glass jar this way right to the top, seal and leave near a sunny window. The syrup will be ready when all the plant material has broken down. Strain through a cloth, bottle and store.

Coltsfoot stimulates the appetite and works as an expectorant, particularly for a hoarse cough. Add 1 teaspoon of dried coltsfoot leaves to 1 cup of almost boiling water. Cover and leave to infuse for 10 minutes. Strain and sweeten if you like. Drink up to two cups per day – as hot as possible.

Linden flowers are well known to induce perspiration and ease muscle aches. Linden flower tea has long been used in the treatment of cold and flu, it also helps ease a sore throat and coughs. Apart from that it is often drunk because it tastes great. Add 1 teaspoon dried linden flowers to 1 cup of almost boiling water, cover and leave for 10 minutes to infuse. Drink twice daily.

Plantain eases coughs and acts as an expectorant. Mild but effective enough to be great for children in the form of a syrup. Plantain tea is made by adding 1 teaspoon of dried plantain to 1 cup of almost boiling water, covering and leaving for 10 minutes to infuse. Three cups of the sweetened tea should be sipped throughout the day.

Onions are often used in the treatment of coughs. You can add a peeled onion to 500ml/1 pint of water and simmer for 15 minutes. Sweeten this brew with brown sugar or honey and drink this cough remedy hot.

Or, I personally like to roughly chop a small onion, put it in a glass jar and cover with honey. Seal the jar and leave overnight. The next day you have a strong onion honey of which you take 1 tablespoon several times a day. Not the best taste, but very effective.

CONSTIPATION

There is nothing worse than not being able to "go" for a few days. If this is the case try eating dried fruit e.g. dried apricots which are well known to stimulate the bowel. Pear juice works well too.

Or you could dissolve 1 tablespoon of honey into 1 cup of warm water and drink this on an empty stomach.

A glass of celery juice daily to encourages a sluggish bowel and helps remove toxins from the body.

CUTS/SMALL WOUNDS

A compress made from plantain juice aids the healing of sprains, ulcers and minor wounds.

Bruise fresh woodruff leaves and apply to slow healing wounds to encourage the healing process.

The fine membrane between layers of onion makes a very effective antiseptic dressing. Apply wounds, cuts or burns and cover with a bandage.

Putting toothpaste on small cuts instantly stops the bleeding.

CHOLESTEROL

To treat high cholesterol drink an infusion made from 3 cloves of garlic, 2 pinches of lavender and 3 pinches of sage. Add 1 cup of almost boiling water, cover and leave to steep for 10 minutes. Drink twice daily.

DANDRUFF

For the treatment of dandruff and to encourage hair growth, add two handfuls of fresh stinging nettles to 600ml/1pint of boiling water. Cover and leave to cool. When cold strain and use the resulting liquid as a hair rinse, massaging it well into the scalp.

Try this effective and cheap treatment: Dissolve one handful of salt in lukewarm water and use this to thoroughly rinse the hair after it has been washed.

Washing hair with an infusion made from birch leaves is excellent against dandruff as well.

DENTAL/TEETH

Drink a sherry glass of blueberry juice daily to ease bleeding gums.

Gargling with astringent oak bark tea on an hourly basis will ease gum inflammation and infection. Add 2 teaspoons of oak bark to 1 cup of water. Bring it to the boil, then gently simmer for 15 minutes. Use this decoction as a gargle when needed, do not swallow.

Bleeding gums can be treated by rubbing teeth and gums with fresh or dried sage leaves.

Chewing cloves – A very old remedy for toothache is to chew a clove with the affected tooth. This will reduce pain and inflammation.

An even older and somewhat unusual remedy for toothache is to inhale a pinch of powdered chalk into the nostril on the same side as the pain. As crazy as it sounds, it is really supposed to work. No one knows why.

Chewing sage leaves daily will brighten teeth as will brushing with baking soda every once in a while.

Another unusual remedy for toothache is to squash a clove of garlic, wrap in a bit of cloth and insert into ear on the side of the pain.

Rub left over lemon rind on your teeth and gums to whiten and strengthen them. Eating an apple with the skin has the same effect of disinfecting the tooth and massages the gum.

To remove plaque and tartar, squash a ripe strawberry, apply to toothbrush and use to brush teeth.

DETOX

Stinging nettles tea detoxifies the blood and is an excellent overall blood purifier. To make the tea add 1 teaspoon of dried nettle leaves to 1 cup of almost boiling water, cover and leave to infuse for 10 minutes. Drink 2 – 3 times a day.

Watercress is often used fresh in salads. Its high vitamin content also makes it a favourite sandwich filling. The dried herb is an effective treatment for water retention, skin disorders and liver dysfunction. Watercress tea is a diuretic and blood purifier. Add 1 teaspoon of dried watercress leaves to 1 cup of almost boiling water, cover and leave to infuse for 10 minutes. Drink one cup, preferably unsweetened, in the morning.

Coltsfoot and the common daisy (Bellis perennis) also called lawn daisy are both excellent blood purifiers. They can be taken individually or mixed together. Mixing the dried flowers give it a very appealing aroma. Add 2 teaspoons of dried herb to 1 cup of almost boiling water, cover and leave to infuse for 5 minutes. Drink up to two cups per day – as hot as possible.

Drinking an infusion made from dandelion leaves or root twice a day will help the gall bladder, strengthen the liver, clean the body via the kidneys and if you add meadowsweet it will also aid the stomach as well. Add 2 teaspoons of dried herb to 1 cup of water. Bring to the *boil, cover and leave to infuse for 10 minutes. Drink a cup morning and evening after meals.*

A glass of celery juice daily to encourages a sluggish bowel and helps remove toxins from the body.

Juniper berries are a well known remedy. They act as a diuretic, drive toxins from the blood and encourage digestion. A tea made from the berries is very useful in the treatment of urinary inflammations, bladder disorders and water retention. Add one teaspoon of bruised dried berries to 1 cup of water, bring to the boil, cover and infuse for 10 minutes. Strain and drink a cup 3 times a day.

Woodruff tea is an effective herb for liver dysfunction, removing toxins and regulating blood circulation. Add 1 teaspoon of dried herb to 1 cup of almost boiling water, cover and leave to infuse for 10 minutes. Drink one cup after the evening meal.

DIGESTION/TUMMY

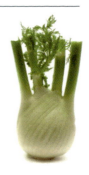

The starch in cooked potatoes soothes a stomach ache. Eating some fresh mashed potato or a mild potato soup is good for you and eases inflammation.

A tea made from aniseed stimulates the appetite, eases stomach aches and helps with bloating. Add 1 teaspoon of bruised seeds to 1 cup of water, bring to the boil, cover and leave off the heat to infuse for 10 minutes.

Fennel can be used raw or steamed to treat digestive disorders. It also has a high content of Vitamin C.

Stomach aches, cramps and inflammations can be soothed with unsweetened chamomile tea. Add 2 teaspoons of chamomile flowers to 1 cup of almost boiling water, cover and leave to infuse for 10 minutes.

Caraway eases bloating and strengthens the digestive system. It is a warming remedy that is especially effective against stomach cramps. Add 1 teaspoon of bruised seeds to 1 cup of water, bring to the boil, cover and leave off the heat to infuse for 10 minutes. Drink at meal times.

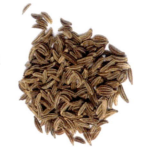

Sage helps treat stomach and bowel dysfunction. It also eases diarrhoea. Add 1 teaspoon of dried sage leaves to 1 cup of almost boiling water, cover and leave to infuse for 10 minutes. Drink a cup before meal times to ease digestion.

DIARRHOEA

Bananas normalise colonic functions in the large intestine to absorb large amounts of water for proper bowel movements.

Fresh mashed potato (without milk or butter) helps prevent the fermentative process in the intestines and helps the growth of friendly bacteria in the digestive tract.

When diarrhoea is first suspected, peel and grate two apples and eat straight away. Repeat every hour. Apples that are not over ripe contain pectins which encourage the removal of toxins which irritate the intestines.

Acute diarrhoea can be eased with a mushy wheat flour remedy. Stir flour into 1 cup of boiled water until you get a thick mush. Take a tablespoon hourly.

A small teaspoon of grated nutmeg will send diarrhoea packing quickly. Unfortunately it tastes rather ghastly.

Strawberry leaves are effective against jaundice and diarrhoea. Add 1 teaspoon of strawberry leaves to 1 cup of almost boiling water, cover and leaves to infuse for 10 minutes. Drink 2 – 3 unsweetened cups a day.

EARS

Built up wax can be treated by first using warmed olive oil as ear drops (35° Celsius = 95° Fahrenheit) for a few days, then rinse the softened wax plug out with lukewarm chamomile tea.

Ease acute ear ache by inserting a clove of garlic into the affected ear.

Wrap freshly cut onion slices in a dry cloth; place this onto the affected ear. After a very short while the onion warms and begins to break down. The pain disappears as the onion "pulls out the pain".

EYES

Treat swollen eyelids and eye strain with chamomile tea. Soak some cotton wool in lukewarm chamomile tea, place on closed eye lids and leave for 10 minutes.

For sensitive or tired eyes you can use eye washes made from blueberries, or linden flowers to ease reddening and itchiness. To make take a handful of flowers, add to 1 cup of almost boiling water, cover and leave for 10 minutes. Strain and use the liquid to make warm compresses for the eyes.

FATIGUE/TIREDNESS

Feeling tired and flat? Try some minted milk made with 1tablespoon of dried mint and 1cup of almost boiling milk - leave to infuse for 5 minutes then strain and drink by taking slow sips.

Nettle juice contains many minerals, especially iron. It is also full of vitamins which will increase your energy levels. Chop whole plants and soften in water for 24 hours. Press through a juicer for a concentrated energy hit.

FISH BONES

Lemon juice softens fish bones. If you have swallowed a fish bone, slowly sip some dilute lemon juice. The bone will soften and stop irritating.

Caution: In some cases a doctor's visit may be advised, especially when it affects children. Better safe than sorry.

FROSTBITE

Add a decoction of Horse Chestnuts to your bath. Also useful for piles and blood circulation issues - chop up the Chestnuts, add to water, bring to the boil, cover and leave to steep for 10 minutes. Add decoction to bath (or footbath or wash basin).

GOUT

Celeriac is useful for gout and rheumatism. Chop up two bulbs cover with water and bring to the boil, cover and gently simmer for 20 minutes. Drink the cooled decoction throughout the day.

Juniper berries are another folk remedy used for the treatment of gout and rheumatism. Add 1 or 2 teaspoons of freshly crushed, dried juniper berries to 1 cup of water, bring to a gentle boil and simmer, covered, for 15 minutes. Drink one cup morning and evening.

Caution: Do not use juniper berries when pregnant.

A decoction of walnut leaves is an effective remedy for gout and purifying the blood. Add a handful of leaves to 1litre/2 pints of water, bring to the boil, cover and gently simmer for 12 minutes. Drink 2 – 3 cups daily. Sweeten with honey if desired.

HAEMORRHOIDS (PILES)

Horse chestnut decoction of the spiky husk as well as the fruit can be used as a wash or added to a full bath increases blood circulation to the area immersed and eases the discomfort of haemorrhoids. Cover 1 kilo/2.2 lbs of chopped husks and nuts with water and bring briefly to the boil, cover and turn off heat. Leave for 30 minutes then add strained liquid to bath water.

HEADACHES

Lemon balm tea helps with colds, headaches and dizziness. Add 1 teaspoon dried lemon balm to 1 cup of almost boiling water, cover and leave for 10 minutes to infuse. Drink twice daily.

Caffeine has been known to dilate blood vessels which can help treat headaches. Try this 'special' coffee said to work wonders. Brew a strong cup of coffee, add the juice of a lemon and drink unsweetened.

Not sure why, but quite often drinking a cup of meaty broth, rich in salt eases a headache.

If the headache is due to tension caused by teeth grinding or generally keeping tense around the jaw, chewing fresh parsley is going to ease the tension as long as you do it at the onset of your headache.

Throw a handful of aniseeds onto glowing coals. Inhaling the smoke through the nose will ease a tension headache.

When you first notice flickering in your vision (aura) eat an apple straight away to keep a migraine at bay.

Treat a migraine with an onion compress placed on the forehead. Slice fresh onions and place on a clean cotton. Wrap into a thin parcel to make the compress.

Similarly, a compress of sliced raw potatoes, sprinkled with pepper applied to the forehead for an hour is said to work very well to hold off a migraine as well.

HICCUPS

Apple cider vinegar is very useful in the treatment of hiccups. Put a few drops onto a cube of sugar and slowly let it dissolve in your mouth.

HOARSENESS

A quick remedy is to whisk up two raw eggs with a little brandy and sipping this a little at a time. Make sure you trust the source of your eggs because I didn't include a remedy for salmonella poisoning in the book.

Wrap a compress of warmed, chopped onion around the throat.

Coltsfoot eases coughs and hoarseness. Add 1teaspoon of chopped coltsfoot to 1 cup of almost boiling water, cover and leave for 10 minutes. Strain, sweeten with honey and drink up to 2 cups daily – as hot as possible.

INFECTIONS

St John's Wort oil is very effective against inflammation and infections. It is also used to treat livestock. Add flowers to cold pressed oil, leave for 3 weeks. Strain well; pour into bottles, label and store.

INDIGESTION/HEARTBURN

Heartburn is eased by slowly chewing a raw piece of potato, a few sips of milk or a spoonful of raw sauerkraut.

The next time that you have indigestion problems, take 1 tablespoon of apple cider vinegar, and follow with a glass of water and be amazed.

INSOMNIA

People are open to all sorts of remedies to ensure a good night's sleep. Here are some of the more unusual, but harmless ones:

Get up and wet your belly button with water, then return to bed to sleep.

Comb or brush your hair for 10 minutes before retiring. This is meant to be a very calming and relaxing activity.

Heat a large cup of milk with a peeled onion, but do not boil. Drink 30 minutes before bedtime.

Some people like a warm bath before bed, others prefer a cold splash of water under the under arms.

A tea made from apple skins is meant to induce sleep. Add dried apple skins to water and bring to a boil. Simmer for 10 minutes, sweeten to taste and drink 2 to 3 cups during the evening.

Now for some of the more common remedies for insomnia:

Valerian is well known to help insomniacs. You can choose to drink a cup of valerian tea or take a few drops of tincture before bed.

Valerian can also be used in a calming bath. Chop or grind 75g/2 ½ oz dried valerian root, add to 2 litres/4 pints of water, bring to the boil and simmer for 5 minutes. Cover and leave to infuse for 20 minutes. Add to the evening bath.

Hops tea is a traditional sleeping aid. Add 2 teaspoons of chopped hops flowers to 1 cup of almost boiling water, cover and leave for 15 minutes. Strain, and drink one cup 30 minutes before bedtime. Drinking hops tea during day will contribute to general relaxation. **Caution:** If sleeplessness is due to depression or low mood disorders please choose a different remedy as hops can make things worse.

Lavender is great in a tea, bath or in a pillow to lend its relaxing aroma to your bedtime routine. For the bath brew a handful of lavender flowers for 15 minutes before straining and adding it to the bathwater.

Add 2 teaspoons of lavender flowers to 1 cup of almost boiling water, cover and leave for 5 minutes. Strain, and drink 1 or 2 cups during the evening.

If insomnia is caused by restlessness, sweet woodruff tea is a well known muscle relaxant.

NAILS

Ingrown nails can be trimmed after wrapping the affected digit in an oil soaked rag overnight. It will be very soft making cutting much easier. Any cooking oil will work.

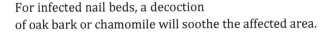

For infected nail beds, a decoction of oak bark or chamomile will soothe the affected area.

NERVES

Valerian is well known to calm the nerves. You can choose to drink a cup of valerian tea or take a few drops of tincture.

The very act of taking a bath can be very soothing but adding herbs with relaxing and calming properties can take it to another level altogether.

Valerian makes a calming bath. Chop or grind 75g/2½ oz dried valerian root, add to 2 litres/4 pints of water, bring to the boil and simmer for 5 minutes. Cover and leave to infuse for 20 minutes. Add to the evening bath. The same can be done with 90ml/3floz of valerian tincture, but it is not as effective as the decoction.

Linden flowers added to a bath lift depression and calm nervousness. Simmer a handful of linden flowers in 1 lire/2 pints of water for 15 minutes, cover and leave to infuse for another 10 minutes. Strain and add to the bathwater.

Rosemary is also great for the nerves, but it also invigorates. Add 100gr/3½ oz rosemary leaves to 3 litres boiling water, cover and leave to infuse for 20 minutes. Strain and add to bathwater.

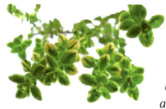
A bath made with thyme flowers can ease nervous exhaustion. Add 100gr/3½ oz thyme leaves and flowers to 2 litres/4 pints boiling water. Cover and leave to infuse for 15 minutes. Strain and add to bathwater.

NIGHTSWEATS

Sage has long been used to battle excessive sweating. A sage infusion can be used as a skin wash or added to bathwater. For the skin wash add 1 teaspoon of chopped sage leaves to 1 cup of almost boiling water, cover and leave for 10 minutes. Strain before use.

NIPPLES

Grated carrots applied directly to cracked nipples will heal and soothe the pain.

RHEUMATISM

*A bath made from hayflowers (*Flores graminis*) is a traditional remedy for rheumatism and rheumatic disorders. Add 2 handfuls of dried hayflowers to 2 litres/4 pints of water, bring to* the boil then simmer for 10 minutes. Strain and use to bathe affected areas.

To treat gout or rheumatism, boil 2 celeriac bulbs in water until cooked out. Strain and squeeze through muslin. Drink this juice over a few days.

A mustard plaster eases a number of back issues such as sciatica, neuralgia, joint inflammation and rheumatic pain. Quantities for the mustard paste will depend on the size of plaster required. Use a piece of cotton or linen cloth at least twice the size required. Grind mustard seeds (be aware that black are the hottest), then add 4 times as much all purpose flour and enough cool water to make a paste. Spread paste onto half the fabric, fold over, if too wet add another layer of cloth, once placed on the affected area this will increase blood circulation, perspiration and heat. Do not let the paste touch bare skin, and do not use for longer than 30 minutes. Remove and wash well with warm water.

Folk medicine also utilises juniper berries to treat rheumatic disorders and gout. Add 1 or 2 teaspoons of freshly crushed, dried juniper berries to 1 cup of water, bring to a gentle boil and simmer, covered, for 15 minutes. Drink one cup morning and evening. **Caution:** Do not use juniper berries when pregnant.

An old remedy for arthritis is to boil some cabbage leaves, cooling them slightly and wrapping the affected area in the warm leaves. This is then covered with a towel.

SORE THROAT

A sore throat is often soothed by gargling. Some effective gargles to be found in the pantry are: Sage tea, chamomile tea and blueberry tea. Sage tea is also used to ease the discomfort of tonsillitis/strep throat.

Drinking linden flower tea will encourage perspiration and loosen up a cramped throat.

Make your tea by adding 1 teaspoon of chopped herb to 1 cup of almost boiling water. Cover and leave to infuse for 10 minutes. Strain and use as desired.

SKIN

Blisters on hands and feet will heal faster with a soft cloth, soaked in alcohol wrapped around the affected area and left over night.

Brewer's yeast, taken daily will prevent skin imperfections, make it smooth and rosy.

Cracked skin on the hands can be treated by soaking a soothing milk bath. Add 3 drops of vegetable oil to warm milk and soak hands for 15 minutes. With regular treatment any redness will recede and hands will return to be smooth and soft.

You can also just rub cooking oil into your hands on a regular basis.

Comfrey root is very useful for the care and treatment of sensitive and irritated skin. Add 2 teaspoons of chopped comfrey root to 1 cup of water. Bring to the boil, cover and simmer for 15 minutes. Soak a cloth in the strained liquid and use as a compress on the affected area.

For dry skin, make a mask out of strawberries, honey and yoghurt. Mix everything together, apply to the face and leave for 15 minutes. Rinse off with tepid water then dab dry.

A parsley poultice soother skin irritations and eases infections.

Plantain juice is a potent treatment for acne and other skin imperfections. Wash and juice plantain leaves. Take 1 tablespoon 3 times a day .

A decoction of walnut leaves applied to the skin will soothe mild inflammations. Put 2 teaspoons of chopped walnut leaves and 1 cup of cold water on the heat. Cover and bring to a boil. Leaving the lid on, remove from heat and steep for 10 minutes. Strain and use to soak compresses or skin wash. Not for internal use.

Horsetail is a great remedy for blemished skin and large pores. Add 1 handful of chopped horsetail to 1 cup of boiling water, cover and leave for 10 minutes. Strain and use as a steam bath or cool the liquid to use for a compress.

To combat oily skin put 3 handfuls of chopped horsetail into an old stocking, tie and hang into the bathwater.

Horsetail is also an effective treatment of itchy skin and eczema. Soak 3 tablespoons of chopped horsetail in 1 litre/2 pints of water over night. Next day bring it to the boil for 3 minutes then leave covered for 10 minutes. Strain, then use to bathe affected areas. **Do not drink**!

STRAINS & SPRAINS

Pick yellow arnica petals, cover with alcohol (vodka) and leave in a cool and dark spot for 3 weeks. Strain and use resulting tincture to rub on strains, sprains and bruising.

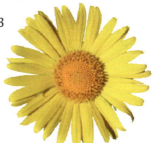

A full arnica bath requires approx. 3 tablespoons of tincture. Or you can make an infusion of 2 teaspoons of dried arnica petals to 1 cup of almost boiling water. Cover and leave steep for 10 minutes. Strain and use resulting liquid to bathe affected areas.

St John's Wort oil is very effective against sprains, strains and other muscle injuries. It is also used to treat livestock. Add flowers to cold pressed oil, leave for 3 weeks. Strain well; pour into bottles, label and store.

A mustard plaster eases a number of back issues such as sciatica, neuralgia, joint inflammation and rheumatic pain. Quantities for the mustard paste will depend on the size of plaster required. Use a piece of cotton or linen cloth at least twice the size required. Grind mustard seeds (black are the hottest), then add 4 times as much plain flour and enough cool water to make a paste. Spread paste onto half the fabric, fold over, if too wet add another layer of cloth, once placed on the affected area this will increase blood circulation, perspiration and heat. Apply to affected area until it heats up (approx 10 minutes). Remove and wash well with warm water. **Caution:** Do not let the paste touch bare skin, and do not use for longer than 30 minutes.

Plantain juice or poultice is a very old remedy for sprains and strains.

SUNBURN

An old but effective home remedy for sunburn is to apply yoghurt or sour cream to the affected area.

Sliced tomatoes placed onto the burned area will soothe and heal the damaged skin.

A tea made from comfrey root makes a soothing remedy for sunburn. Add 2 teaspoons of chopped comfrey root to 1 cup of water. Cover and bring to the boil. Once boiling, remove from the heat and leave to steep for 15 minutes. Soak a cloth in the cooled liquid and place on affected area.

Another home remedy suggests applying stiffly whipped eggwhites to the burned skin. Leave to dry then wash off gently with lukewarm chamomile tea.

WATER RETENTION

While watercress is often used fresh in salads, its high vitamin content also makes it a favourite sandwich filling. The dried herb however, is an effective remedy for water retention, skin disorders and liver dysfunction. Watercress tea is a diuretic and blood purifier. Add 1 teaspoon of dried watercress leaves to 1 cup of almost boiling water, cover and leave to infuse for 10 minutes. Drink 1 cup, preferably unsweetened, in the morning.

WARTS

If you are bothered by warts, apply the milky sap from dandelions directly onto the wart (not the surrounding sensitive skin) twice a day for a few days or until it falls off. The area can be covered with a bandage to keep sap only on the wart.

The sap of fresh fig leaves works in a similar fashion to dandelions.

Apply a fresh slice of garlic to the wart in the morning and evening. Use a bandage to keep in place. Onions work in a similar way with the wart disappearing after about 6 weeks of treatment.

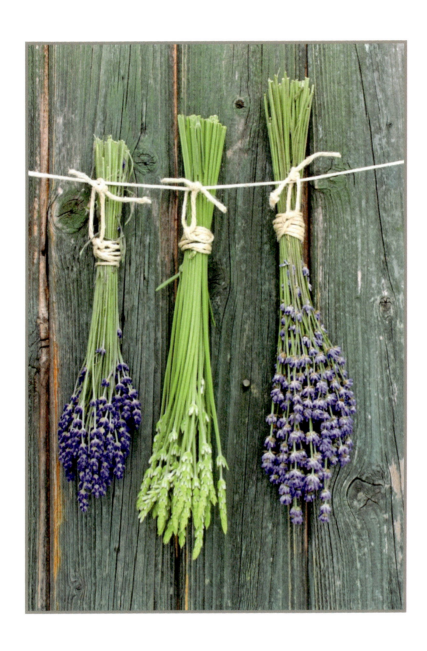

Picking, Drying & Storing

Picking vegetables, fruit and herbs is an ongoing process. Different plants have different requirements, some you can pick at while dormant, others like a good cutting back to produce a second crop.

Here is an overview of harvesting different plant materials.

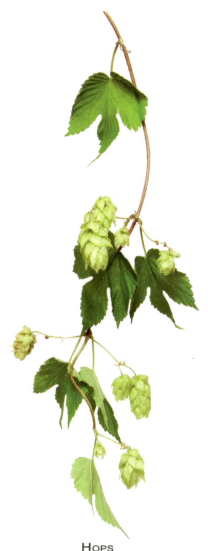

HOPS
Humulus lupulus

PICKING

TIME OF DAY

Choose a fine, sunny morning to do your harvesting, early enough that the heat of the sun has not yet caused the volatile oils to dissipate but late enough that there is no more moisture from dew or rain on the plant. If the plants get too hot you will lose too much goodness and if picked wet they go mouldy before properly dried.

LEAVES

Leaves will be at their most potent before flowering as all the plants energy went into the stems. Once flowers form the energy is shared.

Pick small leafed herbs by the stem and strip them off later. Larger leaves can be picked individually. Only keep the best leaves to dry and store. Dead and discoloured leaves can contribute to the making of compost.

FLOWERS

Flowers should be cut either just before or shortly after opening. They are best while their colour and scent are at their best and before their petals have dropped. Pick flowers individually. Some, like lavender, are picked with a long piece of stem attached whereas others just the actual 'head' is carefully picked off. For some you may wish to strip the petals and for other, often smaller flowers you will want to keep them whole to dry.

SEEDS

Seeds are harvested before they are ready to fall but after they have lost their green colour. They can go from green to ripe very quickly so you have to keep a close eye on them before they start to spread. Collect the whole 'head' and retrieve the individual seeds later. If you think you are going to lose the seeds you can tie some paper or muslin around the 'head' before they are ripe.

ROOTS (RHIZOMES)

Roots are best harvested later in the growing year when the

plant is dormant while leaf growth is at a minimum. When cutting roots you may wish to leave a portion in the ground so the plant can regenerate in spring. Some herbs, like comfrey, don't need much encouragement for regrowth and will return with even the smallest bit of root left in the ground.

BULBS

Bulbs like onion and garlic are dug up in late summer or early autumn. You can usually tell that they are ready for harvest by the green parts above ground having dropped to the ground and turned brown.

BARK

Make sure you don't strip bark from very young trees and do not 'ring bark' which means stripping bark all the way around the trunk. Do not take too much bark from the same tree as this might kill it. Use sharp and clean tools and keep your cuts 1m/3ft above ground. Lastly, do not harvest from endangered or protected species.

WILD FOODS

Be sure the plant you pick is the plant you think it is. Correct identification is vital; your life may depend on it. If you have any doubt, leave them where they are. Check the environment, there is no point picking in areas that are subjected to heavy pollution or exposed to pesticides.

Many wild plants are protected by law; educate yourself about the rules of wildcrafting in your local area. Do not over pick, leave some to spread for future harvest and to maintain growth in the area.

DRYING

To dry your herbs you need to create the right environment. Perfect conditions for drying include a consistently high temperature and low humidity. Sun drying is an age old practice but for herbs it can be detrimental, causing colour loss and losing all important volatile oils as well. You'll want to dry your plant material as quickly as possible before the natural process of decay sets in, but not use excessive heat to speed up the process.

Ovens have been used but the heat tends to be too fierce and there is some anecdotal evidence that microwaves work but, personally, I believe the drying to be uneven. The use of a glass of water to maintain proper microwave conditions also defeats the purpose of keeping humidity low. A dehydrator that circulates the air and has a temperature control works very well.

Ideally you'd have a space that is dry, well aired and where the temperature is consistently between 20–32C/68–90F. Avoid dust and direct sunlight, this will keep your plant material clean and preserve colour.

If your plants are particularly dusty or dirty, or you used chemicals (which I know most of you don't) do wash them. Fill a tub with cold water and dunk your plant material several times to remove any impurities. Lay out on a draining board and pat dry gently between clean tea towels.

LEAVES
If the leaf is very small you may wish to dry some herbs on the stem, where as larger leaves you may wish to dry individually. Spread your leaves out on trays, frames stretched with netting or hang tied in small bunches. Leave enough for air to circulate freely. Drying time varies depending on thickness, moisture content and humidity in the air. The rule of thumb is to dry leaves until they are crisp and crackly to the touch. This process can take anywhere between 3 days to a week.

FLOWERS
If the blooms are quite large, remove the petals to dry. Calendula/Marigold flowers can be dried whole and the petals removed afterwards. Lavender flowers are kept on a long stem and hung tied in bunches to dry.

Like leaves, flowers can be dried on trays or netting but if you need the buds to stay in particularly good shape for decorative purposes then you might wish to dry them upright with stems pushed through wire trays. Leave until flowers are papery and dry.

SEEDS

Pick seed heads with stems attached and make sure they're free from insect life. Tie stems into bunches then invert then into a paper bag (do not use plastic, it attracts moisture) and tie the bag around the seed heads. Hang up and leave to dry in a warm, airy place. Once the seeds are completely dry, clean off any pods or husks.

ROOTS & BARK

Scrub roots and bark thoroughly then chop into small pieces ready for drying. These tougher plant materials require higher drying temperatures and can be dried in the sun. Here the oven can be used quite successfully at a very low temperature and the door left slightly open.

Dried outside on trays or netting it is advised to cover with muslin or the like to keep dust and debris away. The roots/bark is dried when it they snap easily. Overall drying your own is easy. Just remember to keep it warm, dry, clean and don't let the plants touch while drying.

STORING

You've picked and dried your healing harvest and now it's time to store everything properly to make it last.

Realistically you can't beat the classic glass jar for storing dried herbs. It seals well, protects from damp and dust, insects stay out and you can see if anything has gone awry with the contents. Keeping an eye on your herbs is especially important in the first couple of weeks after drying in case there is residual moisture which leads to mould.

Choosing the right jar is not rocket science. It has to be whole, clean and dry. Don't make it too large or too small. Collect all manner of sizes throughout the year so you'll have a wide choice when you need it. Make sure there are no remaining odours from whatever occupied the jar last as this will affect your herbs. Label your jars with common name (maybe even botanical name) and date. Store jars in a cool and dark spot.

Of course a jar is not the only way to store your herbs.

You can preserve your herbs in oil too. I prefer not to use fresh herbs in oil as the moisture content promotes rancidity and then there is the whole botulism issue. I am not sure that there has been a reported case of botulism from infused oils, but the common rule is to use plant material that is completely dried, completely submerged in the oil and which is completely removed before storing for any length of time. If you are planning on using the oil up within a week of making, then you can leave the herbs in – they do look rather pretty.

If you are concerned about the loss of colour and flavour through drying, you could always use freezing as your method of preservation. Frozen herbs are useful for cooking and for use in making beauty products.

TO FREEZE HERBS

If your herbs need cleaning, wash them quickly and dry on kitchen paper. If they are organic and grown free of pollution they won't need washing. Strip leaves and petals from the stems. Lay herbs in single layers and pack them flat in a container or zip-lock bag. Make sure you remove as much air from the bag as possible. Mark your chosen container with the name and date. When you need to remove herbs from the freezer work quickly. You'll want to chop a piece off your herb sheet before it defrosts and goes soggy. I also like to freeze mine in ice cube trays. This allows me little portion sizes to add to my favourite recipes without defrosting too much. You can chop them and freeze straight away or you can blend with a little water and freeze the resulting pulp. Use herbs frozen, don't defrost them first.

Storing your herbal bounty well means that you are able to access the wonderful flavours and health giving properties of herbs all year round.

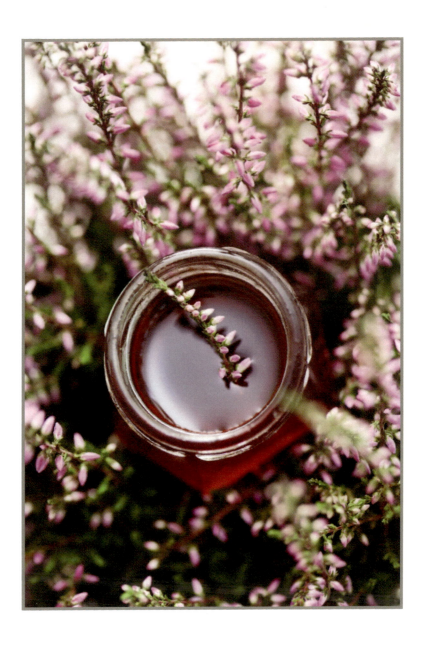

Methods of Preparation

DO YOU KNOW THESE BASE RECIPES?

- Herbal tea
- Infusions
- Decoctions
- Tinctures
- Syrups
- Infused oils
- Creams & Ointments
- Poultice & Compresses

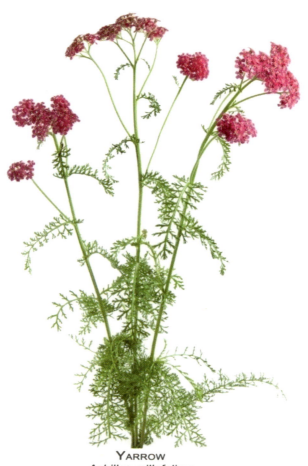

Yarrow
Achillea millefolium

HERBAL TEA

Herbal tea or tisanes are infusions - however a medicinal infusion is a lot stronger than a cup of herbal tea, therefore more of the herb material is needed.

To make herbal tea use 1 teaspoon of dried herb for every cup of almost boiling water. Cover and leave for approximately 10 minutes.

INFUSION

Infusions are made of leaves, flowers, soft seeds and green stems.

30gr/1oz dried herb for every 1 litre/2 pints of almost boiling water. Cover and let infuse for 30 minutes. This formula works on a standard dosage of 3 times daily and makes approximately 3 doses.

DECOCTION

Decoctions require simmering for a long time, opposed to steeping in boiled water like infusions. This means that the materials used in the tea must be crushed beforehand and cut into small pieces suitable for simmering temperatures. This method is just as simple as infusing as it only consists of a few simple steps.

30gr/1oz dried herb for every 1 litre/2 pints cold water which reduces down to approx 750ml/1½ pints. Bring up to heat and simmer gently for up to 30 minutes.

This formula works on a standard dosage and makes approximately 3 doses. Decoctions should be made fresh each day and should be stored in the fridge. It may be sweetened and can be drunk hot or cold.

Tinctures are stronger than water based extractions like infusions or decoctions, as some of the active ingredients in the plant may not be water soluble but will dissolve in alcohol.

A rule of thumb is 1 part herb to 5 parts vodka.

Chop herbs finely, then place into a glass jar. Do not pack them tightly or else the vodka won't be able to get to it all. Add vodka to the herbs. If the vodka does not cover all the plant material add some more until it is all completely submerged.

Put a tight lid on the jar and store for 2 weeks at room temperature. A dark shelf is fine, since tincture does not need light to process. Shake the contents once or twice a day to redistribute the herbs in the alcohol. If you are using powdered herbs, stir them with a spoon every day to keep them from clumping together.

Strain the herb pulp through a coffee filter or some muslin/cheesecloth. I like using two layers of muslin. Squeeze out all of the tincture and discard the left over pulp. Funnel into a sterilised, dark glass bottle. Label and store in a cool, dark place.

The standard dose for tinctures, unless otherwise stated, works on 2ml three times a day. Tinctures should always be taken in a little warm water (or juice if you need to disguise the flavour).

SYRUP

To make a particularly unpleasant herbal remedy more palatable it is sometimes a good idea to sweeten the experience by making a syrup. You can use honey or unrefined sugar or you may even wish to add some glycerine as it keeps a lot longer.

500ml/1pint of infusion or decoction to 500gr/1lb of sugar. Heat gently until all the sugar is dissolved. Store syrup in the fridge for future use.

INFUSED OIL

Pack as much herb material into a clear glass jar as you can and cover with oil (vegetable or olive is fine). Seal tightly with a lid and place in the sun, or another warm place for 2 – 3 weeks. After that, strain the infused oil into a dark glass bottle. The oil is ready for use straight away and if stored away from direct light will last for up to a year. To increase the strength of your infused oil you may repeat the process by packing a jar with new herbs, covering it with the already infused oil and leave again for a few weeks.

MASSAGE OIL

In general, use 10-15 drops of essential oil (less if treating children or those with sensitive skin) 125ml/ ½cup of carrier oil. Make small batches as the effectiveness of essential oils deteriorates quickly.

CREAM

A cream is an emulsion of water with oils which softens and soaks into the skin.

180ml/6floz herbs infused oil, 300ml/10floz warm water, 10g/1/3ozbeeswax (not paraffin), 8 drops essential oil (optional). Combine infused oil and beeswax, and heat mixture just enough to melt the wax. Heat the water in a separate pot until warm – (not hot). Put the warm water into your blender/food processor. With the blender running at low speed, slowly add the oil-wax mixture in a steady stream. Half way through (or thereabouts) you'll see the mixture turn white and thicken. This is the time to add the essential oil, if you are using any. Keep adding oil until all used. Don't turn off the blender until all the water has been well combined.

The mixture will be too thick to pour, so use a spatula to fill your jars while the cream is still warm. Stored at room temperature, this cream will keep for 6 months. If you store it in the fridge (and don't use it with your fingers) it may well last 3 times that long.

OINTMENT

Unlike creams, ointments are not made with water. Also known as salves or balm, these preparations are meant to form a layer on the skin, which makes them perfect for providing protection for such things as nappy rash. Ointments are sometimes made with animal fats but it is more common to use petroleum jelly or beeswax.

250ml/8floz infused oil, 25g/1oz beeswax, 8 drops of essential oil (optional).

Heat the oil and stir gently until the wax just melts. Often this is done in a double boiler. Remove from heat and add essential oil. Stir, then pour into dark glass jars. Let cool. Ointment will keep in a cool, dark place for around 4 months.

POULTICE

A poultice is often used to speed up the healing of wounds and muscle injuries. Either dried or fresh herbs may be used to make a poultice.

Use as much herb material as needed to cover the affected area. In an acute situation you can grab a handful of fresh herb, bruise it and place directly onto the injury. Dried herbs must be made into a paste using hot water.

You can pre prepare poultices in a blender by blending fresh herbs with a little water to make a thick paste. Lay on a large piece of unbleached calico and fold into a parcel. This can be made in varying sizes, frozen in zip lock bags for times when the herbs are not available and heated up when needed. Once heated, you can apply the whole parcel to the affected area.

Compresses are similar to poultices but utilise only a liquid extract of the required herb. Use a clean cloth made of a natural fibre (linen, cotton or gauze) and soak it in a hot decoction or infusion. Place on the affected area as hot as bearable. Since heat activates the healing properties it is a good idea to place a hot water bottle on the area to maintain temperature. If this is impractical you may need to repeat the soaking process whenever the compress cools down.

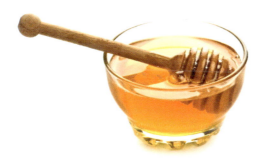

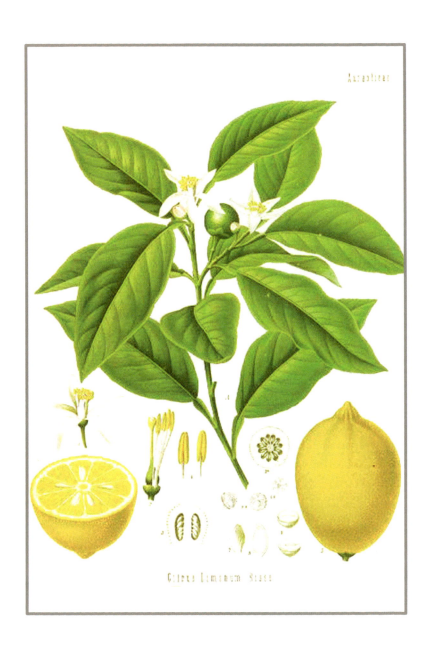

Citrus Limonum Risso

Common/Botanical Names

DO YOU KNOW YOUR URTICA FROM YOUR ALLIUM?

It's useful to know the botanical names for the plants that you use so that you don't accidentally grab one that can have quite dangerous consequences.

This list includes many useful common names you may come across. Common names found in this book are highlighted in **bold**.

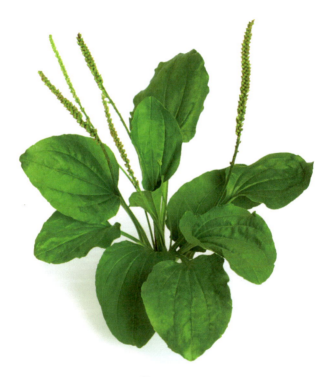

PLANTAIN
Plantago major

Angelica, *Angelica archangelica*

Anise hyssop, *Agastache foeniculum*

Anise, *Pimpinella anisum*

Arnica, *Arnica montana*

Artemisia, *Artemisia spp.*

Basil, Sweet, *Ocimum basilicum*

Bee balm, *Monarda didyma*

Birch, *Betula spp.*

Borage, *Borago officinalis*

Burnet, Salad,*Sanguisorba minor*

Calendula (Pot Marigold), *Calendula officinalis*

Caraway, *Carum carvi*

Catnip, *Nepta cataria*

Chamomile, *Chamaemelum nobile*

Chervil, *Anthriscus cerefolium*

Chives, *Allium schoenoprasum*

Clary sage, *Salvia sclarea*

Clove, *Eugenia caryophyllata*

Coltsfoot, *Tussilago farfara*

Comfrey, *Symphytum officinalis*

Coriander (cilantro), *Coriandrum sativum*

Costmary, *Tanacetum balsamita*

Daisy, Common, *Bellis perennis*

Dandelion, *Taraxacum officinale*

Dill, *Anethum graveolens*

Fennel, *Foeniculum vulgare*

Feverfew, *Tanacetum parthenium*

Garlic, *Allium sativum*

Geranium, Scented, *Pelargonium spp.*

Germander, *Teucrium chamaedrys*

Ginger, *Zingiber officinale*

Hayflowers, *Flores graminis*

Hops, *Humulus lupulus*

Horehound, *Marrubium vulgare*

Horse chestnut, *Aesculus hippocastanum*

Hoseradish, *Armoracia rusticana*

Horsetail, *Equisetum arvense*

Hyssop, *Hyssopus officinalis*

Juniper, *Juniperus communis*

Lavender, *Lavandula angustifolia*

Lemon verbena, *Aloysia triphylla*

Lemon balm, *Melissa officinalis*

Linden, *Tilia cordata*

Lovage, *Levisticum officinale*

Marjoram, *Origanum majorana*

Meadowsweet, *Filpendula ulmarianum*

Mistletoe, *Viscum album*

Mustard Seeds (yellow), *Brassica juncea*

Mustard Seeds (black), *Brassica nigra*

Nasturtium, *Tropaeolum spp.*

Nutmeg, *Myristica fragrans*

Oak bark, *Quercus robur*

Oregano, *Origanum vulgare*

Parsley, *Petroselinum crispum*

Peppermint, *Mentha x piperita*

Plantain, *Plantago lanceolata*

Rosemary, *Rosemarinus officinalis*

Rue, *Ruta graveolens*

Sage, *Salvia officinalis*

Sorrel, *Rumex spp.*

Southernwood, *Artemisia abrotanum*

Spearmint, *Mentha spicata*

St John's Wort, *Hypericum perforatum*

Stinging Nettle, *Urtica dioica*

Summer savory, *Satureja hortensis*

Sweet woodruff, *Galiumodoratum*

Sweet rocket, *Hesperis matronalis*

Tansy, *Tanacetum vulgare*

Tarragon, *Artemisia dracunculus*

Thyme, Common, *Thymus vulgaris*

Valerian, *Valeriana officinalis*

Watercress, *Nasturtium officinale*

Winter savory, *Satureja montana*

Wormwood, *Artemisia absinthium*

Yarrow, *Achillea millefolium*

Bibliography

Braun, Lesley and Marc Cohen. Herbs & Natural Supplements: An evidence-based guide. 2nd ed. Sydney: Elsevier, 2007.

Culpeper, Nicholas. The English Physitian: Or an astrologo-physical discourse of the vulgar herbs of this nation.London: Peter Cole, 1652.

Green, James. The Herbal Medicine-Maker's Handbook: A home manual. Berkeley: Crossing Press, 2000.

Grieve, Maud. A Modern Herbal. New York: Dover, 1971.

Hemphill, John and Rosemary Hemphill. Herbs: Their cultivation and usage. Sydney: Allen & Unwin, 2007.

Hoffmann, David. The Complete Illustrated Holistic Herbal. Shaftesbury: Element Books Ltd, 1996.

Keville, Kathi. Herbs for Health and Healing: A drug-free guide to prevention and cure. Emmaus: Rodale Press Inc, 1996.

Mcvicar, Jekka. New Book of Herbs. London: Dorling Kindersley Limited, 2002.

Ody, Penelope. The Complete Medicinal Herbal. New York: DK Publishing Inc, 1993.

Ody, Penelope. Home Herbal. Australia: Penguin, 1995.

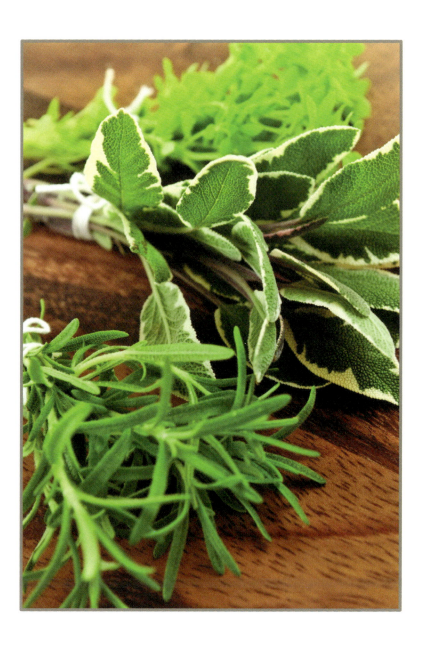

Index

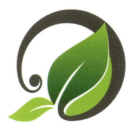

For instant access to the *Herbology On The Go* iPhone app, just use a QR reader on your smartphone to scan the code below.

About the author

Fortunate to have been raised with herbal traditions, Anke Bialas has expanded her knowledge of herbs and their applications over the years, which she now shares with those new to natural health on *Herbology.com.au* She encourages use of herbs in unconventional ways, advocating that even a little bit of nature goes a long way. With a firm believe that herbal health can fit into even the most conventional home, she makes all things herbal appealing to everyone.

Anke is known for her practical, everyday approach to herbal health which led to the creation of the *Herbology At Home* series of guides to herbs and natural health, which provide a convenient reference you can take with you where you need them most.

More titles in the *"Herbology at Home"* series:
Making Herbal Remedies – 2010

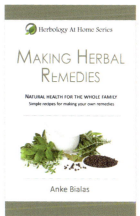 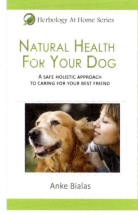

Natural Health For Your Dog – 2011
Connect with Anke online:
Twitter.com/HerbologyAtHome
Facebook.com/Herbology

CPSIA information can be obtained
at www.ICGtesting.com
Printed in the USA
LVIC042214280213
322112LV00010B

* 9 7 8 0 9 8 0 7 6 6 8 5 1 *